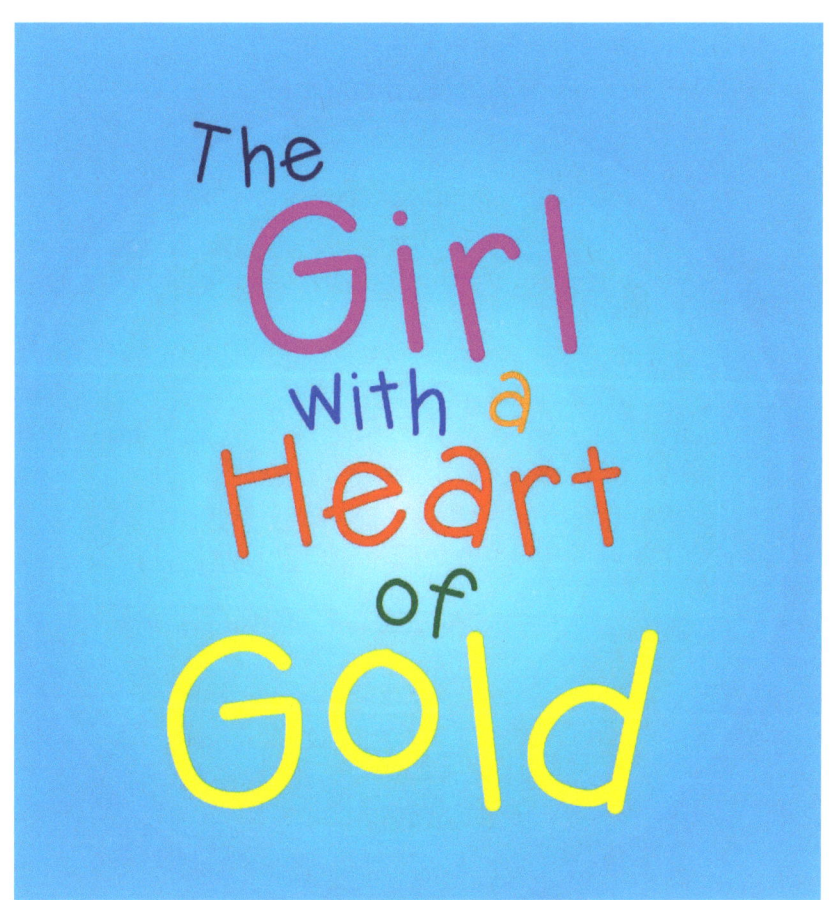

Ieisha Michelle

MY PURPOSE BOOK PUBLISHING
West Covina, California

The Girl with a Heart of Gold
Published by:
My Purpose Book Publishing
West Covina, California
Email: info@thegirlwithaheartofgold.com
Website: www.thegirlwithaheartofgold.com

Ieisha Howell, Publisher
Yvonne Rose / QualityPress.info, Book Packager
Printed Page, Interior & Cover Layout
Cover & Interior Illustrations by Leontre Tabor

ALL RIGHTS RESERVED

No part of this book may be reproduced or transmitted in any form or by any means—electronic or mechanical, including photocopying, recording or by any information storage and retrieval system—without written permission from the authors, except for the inclusion of brief quotations in a review.

The illustrations in this book are the sole property of My Purpose Book Publishing.

Copyright © 2015 by Ieisha Howell
ISBN #: 978-0-9965846-0-9
Library of Congress Control Number: 2015910847

DEDICATION

You lifted me up. You've had me out on a limb, with nothing to hold on to but you. You let me go out and try to figure it out, to only turn around and come back to you. You uplifted me. You always gave me a choice. It took time to build what we have. It took time to let go and trust you. You helped in building my character. You helped in showing me Gods love. You helped in making me the woman I am today. You are the key to life, my life. I put my entire life in your hands. You put the fire under my feet, day after day, when I didn't want to move. You were there when I thought I was alone. At my lowest you were there. At my highest you were there. And through it all, you never left me. Really, you gave me no choice. At times, all I had was you…. FAITH…I thank you. Without you I would have truly been lost. But today, I AM FOUND.

ACKNOWLEDGEMENTS

To my parents, my heroes, my sister and nephew, my inspiration and light… Thank you. My extended family and friends who prayed and uplifted me daily and pushed me until I stepped out on faith. Popo, you will always and forever be my ray of light, shining down on me. Larrance, thank you for all you do, and for giving me something to smile about every day. I'm forever grateful for you all!!

A special thank you to Dr. Ronnie Williams of Kaiser Fontana and his awesome nurse Margarita who regardless of how bad I felt would always put a smile on my face. Thank you for caring!

XOXO,

Ieisha

LOVE, LAUGH, LIVE

INTRODUCTION

Have you ever felt like sometimes you don't fit in? Or, have you ever realized that as much as you love your parents, and they would give their very lives to save yours that they in moments don't understand your specific struggles? It's hard being a kid with visible differences, invisible setbacks and handicaps. Everyone doesn't quite "get it". Let's face it, kids can be cruel sometimes, but I am here to say, it doesn't matter what you are faced with, you can overcome anything. This is the first book of many by the author, Ieisha Howell. It is not only for children suffering from asthma, but all children that have to contend with childhood afflictions, such as: obesity, dyslexia, wearing glasses, autism, battling cancer, loss of limbs; or kids who sometimes, just don't fit in. The girl with the heart of gold is their voice. The author states boldly that her diagnosis hasn't changed, she still has asthma; but what has changed is her heart. Asthma no longer controls her destiny, but rather she controls it. She has overcome what made her different from other kids, to become the difference for all children who are faced with struggles. The Girl with a Heart of Gold is about learning how to breathe; because it's different for us.

This book has been something that has been echoing in my heart for many years. I'd find myself walking in the mall, and have a waking vision of me actually writing the book, and sharing my story. At night, while I was sound asleep God would wake me up with words to write, and I'd know, "Ieisha, get to writing!" However, for years I was afraid to write the book, and never put the pen to the paper. I'd find myself gratifying the desire by writing inspirational quotes, and all types of poetry, but forgetting to write what was burning in my heart.

I can even remember back in junior high, that my girlfriends would have me write poems for them to give to their crushes. As a matter of fact I would write on books, tear out scratch pieces of paper, use a sturdy napkin, just to doodle all the time. There was one problem, everything I wrote only lived inside the dozens of journals stored safely in my room, never to be read or seen by anyone except me. Often, I would open up a little, via social media, and post a little something here or there, but that was the most I could bring myself to do at the time.

Eventually people started to take notice of my post, and I started hearing people tell me, "You know you should write a book or something." Being a woman of faith, I prayed for guidance, and soon after God answered my prayers by sending a good friend by the name of Micha to encourage me to just do it, and use the secret gift God had given me. So that's exactly what I did. That same night like so many nights before, God woke me up again, but this time I opened up my laptop and started writing what later became The Girl with a Heart of Gold. Let me be transparent, for a little while after writing this book, that same nervousness reappeared, and again I sat, having no idea where to start in getting this book out to the world.

I asked around, but that really didn't get me anywhere, because if I am honest, I can say that I wasn't putting my whole heart into the effort. As God would have it, one day my good friend Shante called me, and told me she had a word of encouragement for me, and that's what pushed me to finally do this. After all the years of being awakened out of my sleep, conquering the fear, finally putting pen to paper, I made the commitment to get this book published. I said to myself, *Enough is enough Ieisha, no more fear!*

There was a girl named Michelle, who had a great big heart. Everywhere she went she shined. She made everyone laugh, and was always the life of the party. Even though she had a heart of gold, she had bad lungs. And that really scared her. Michelle had asthma, a condition where her lungs made it hard to breath. Michelle didn't like telling her friends about her asthma because some of the kids would act weird when she got sick and had to go to the hospital. They would laugh and talk about her like she was contagious.

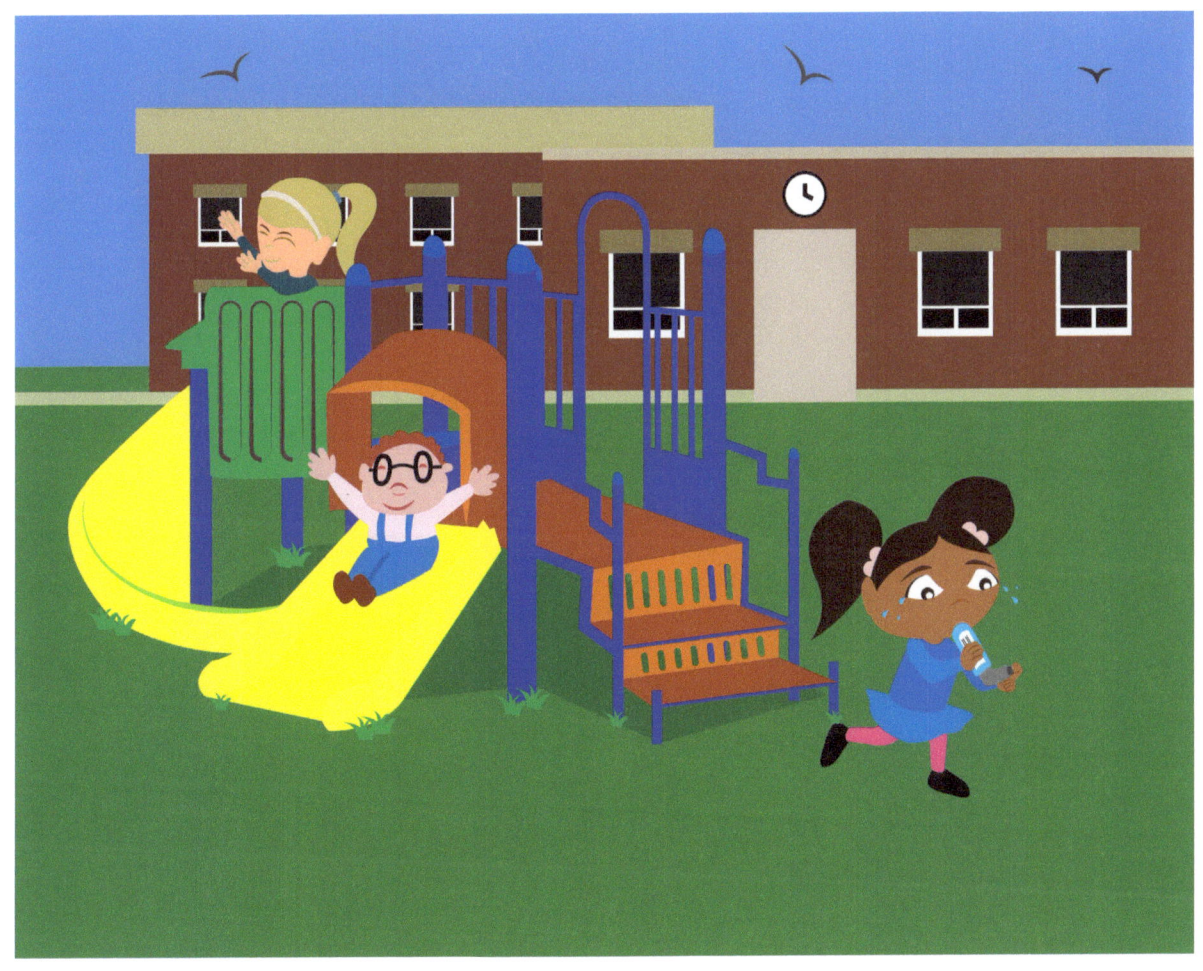

Some of the kids even thought Michelle was faking it when she had to stop playing and take her inhaler. This made her sad and embarrassed and she always felt like she didn't fit in. So she would hide when she had to take her inhaler.

Michelle would want to play with her friends at recess so bad but she was scared she would have an asthma attack. So she would sit out at recess by herself.

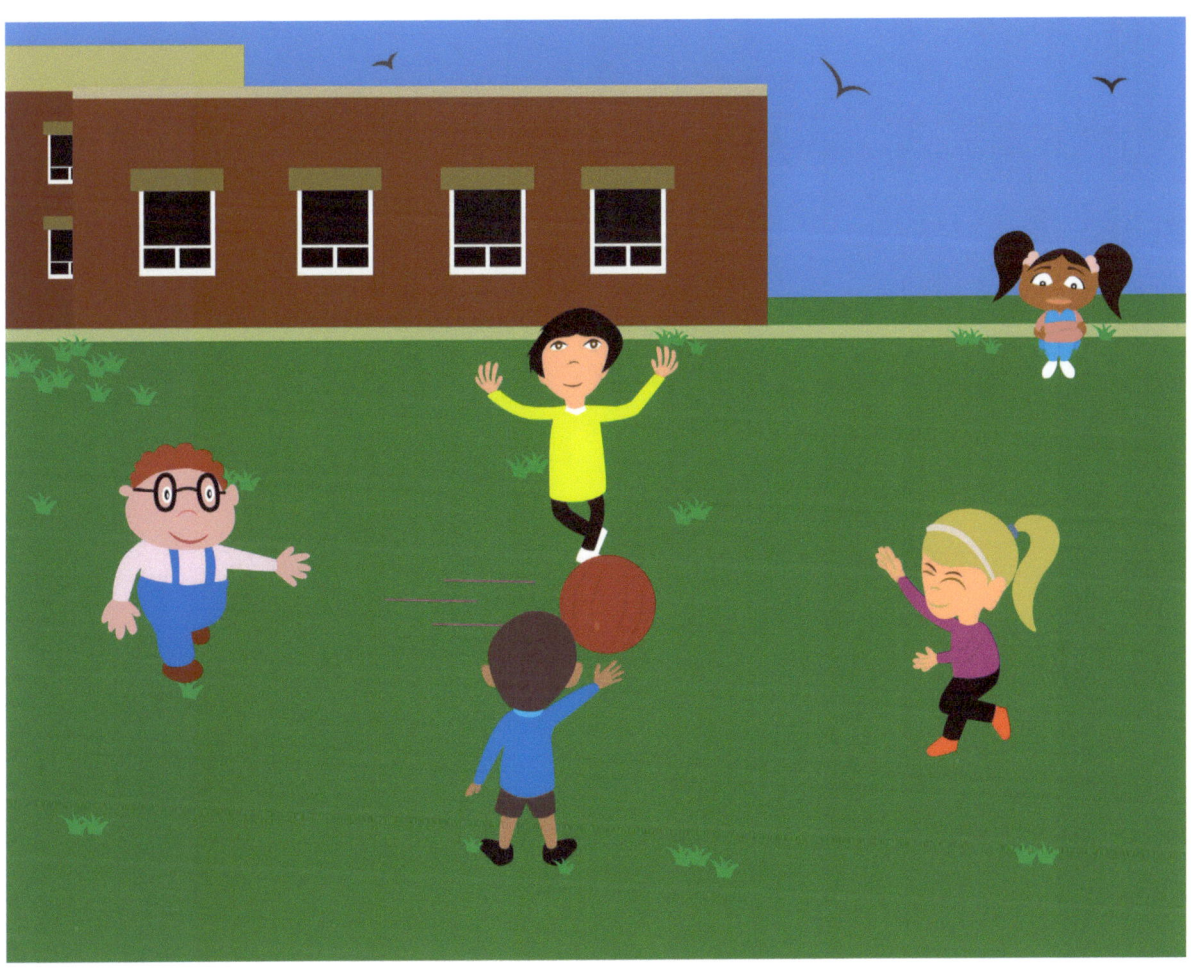

Michelle would get home from school and see her brothers and sisters playing in the front yard every day but would go color her books instead, because she just knew if she started playing she would get an attack.

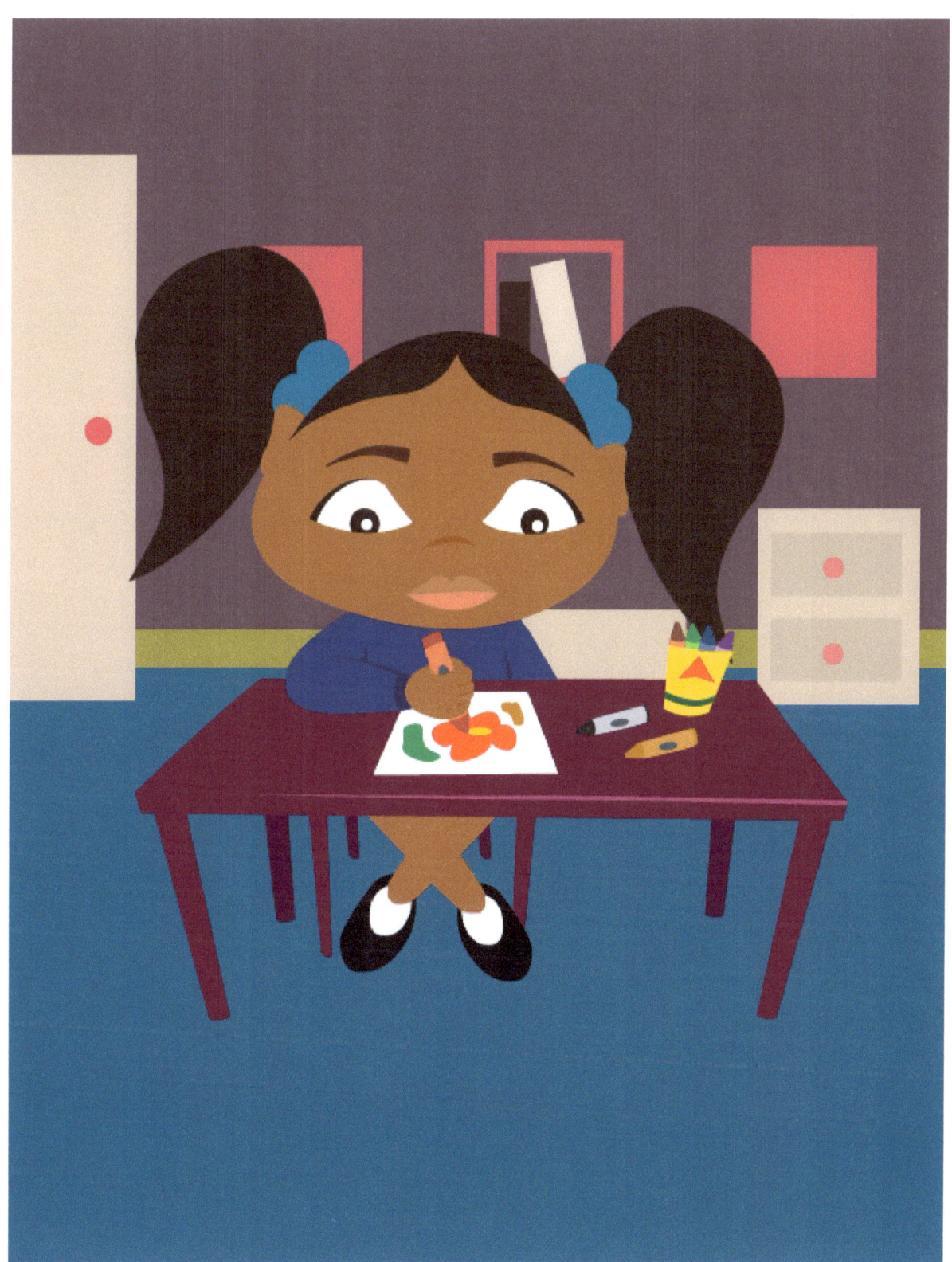

The next day Michelle had to go to the doctor's to check up on her asthma. While she was in the waiting room with her mom, Michelle spotted two of her friends from school, Bryce and Tristan.

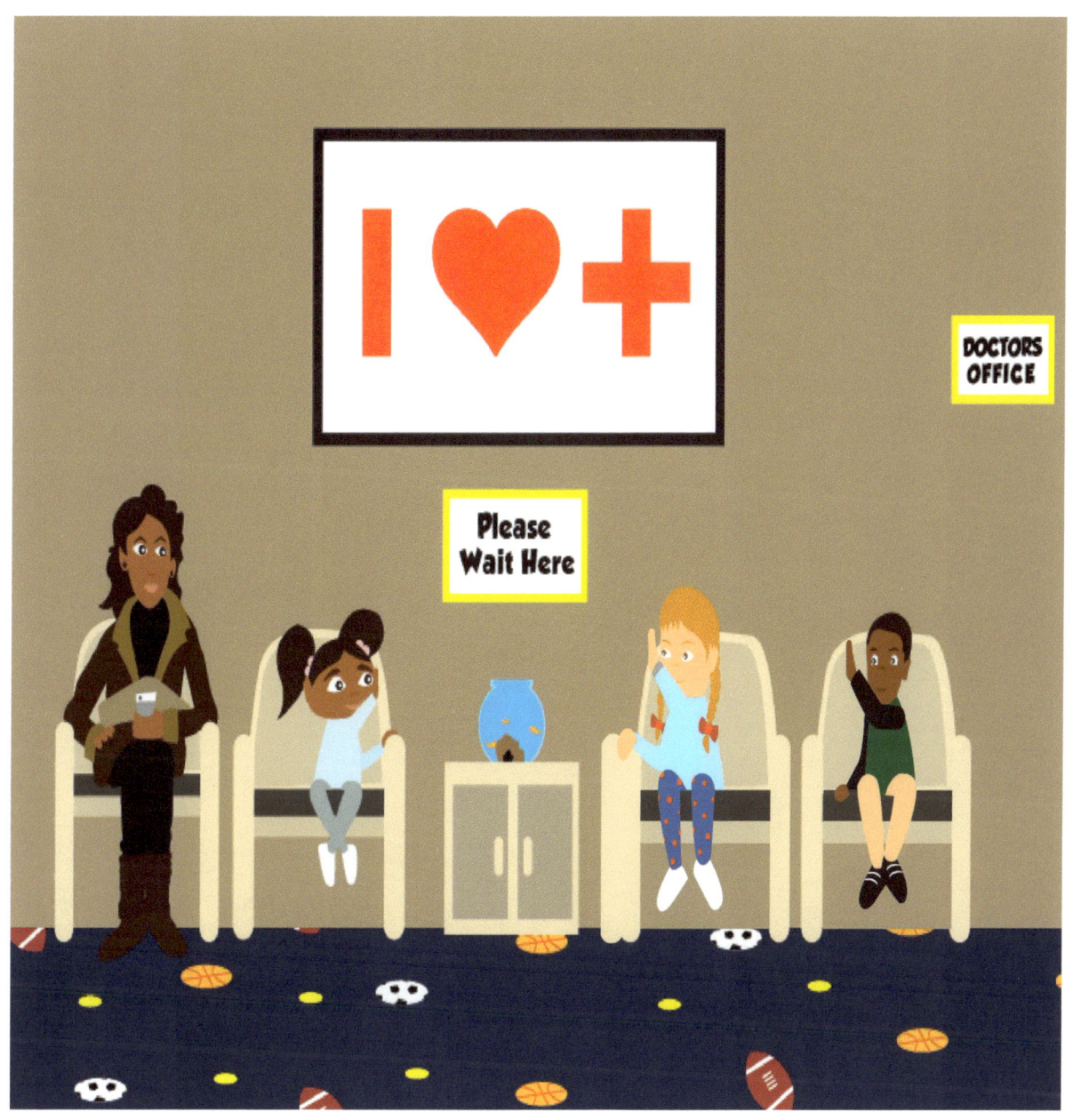

"Hey I didn't know you guys had asthma. So do I," Michelle said to her friends.

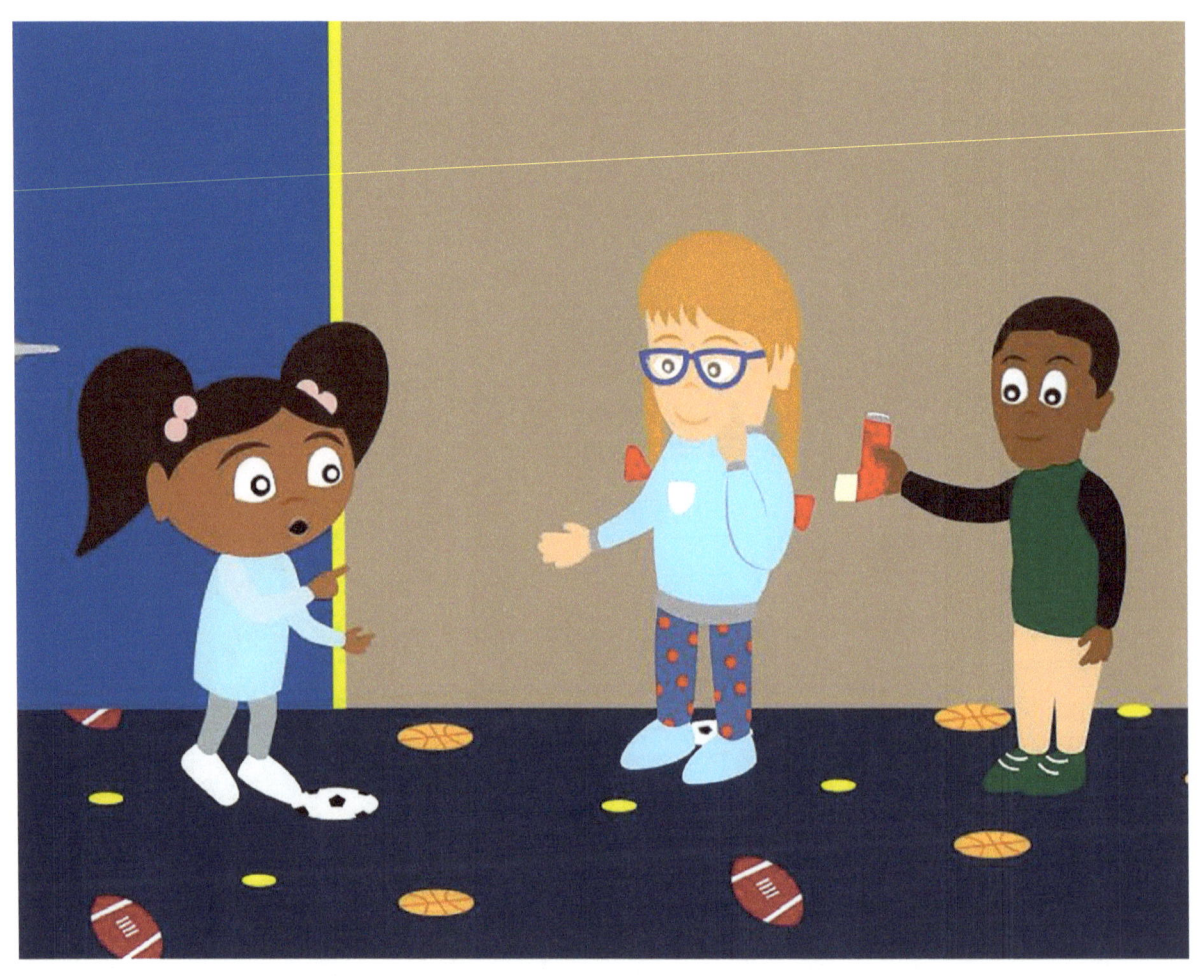

"I've had asthma since I was 5," said Bryce. "And I'm here for my eye appointment," said Tristan.

When Michelle and her mom were leaving the doctor's office, Michelle's friend Bryce invited her to his soccer game. Michelle agreed, but she was so confused. She didn't understand how Bryce was able to play soccer with asthma.

Michelle's mom took her along with her brother and sister to Bryce's game that weekend. Michelle sat there in amazement because Bryce was playing just as hard as the other players and she didn't see him take his pump at all during the game. After the game, Michelle ran to Bryce in excitement asking him how he did it.

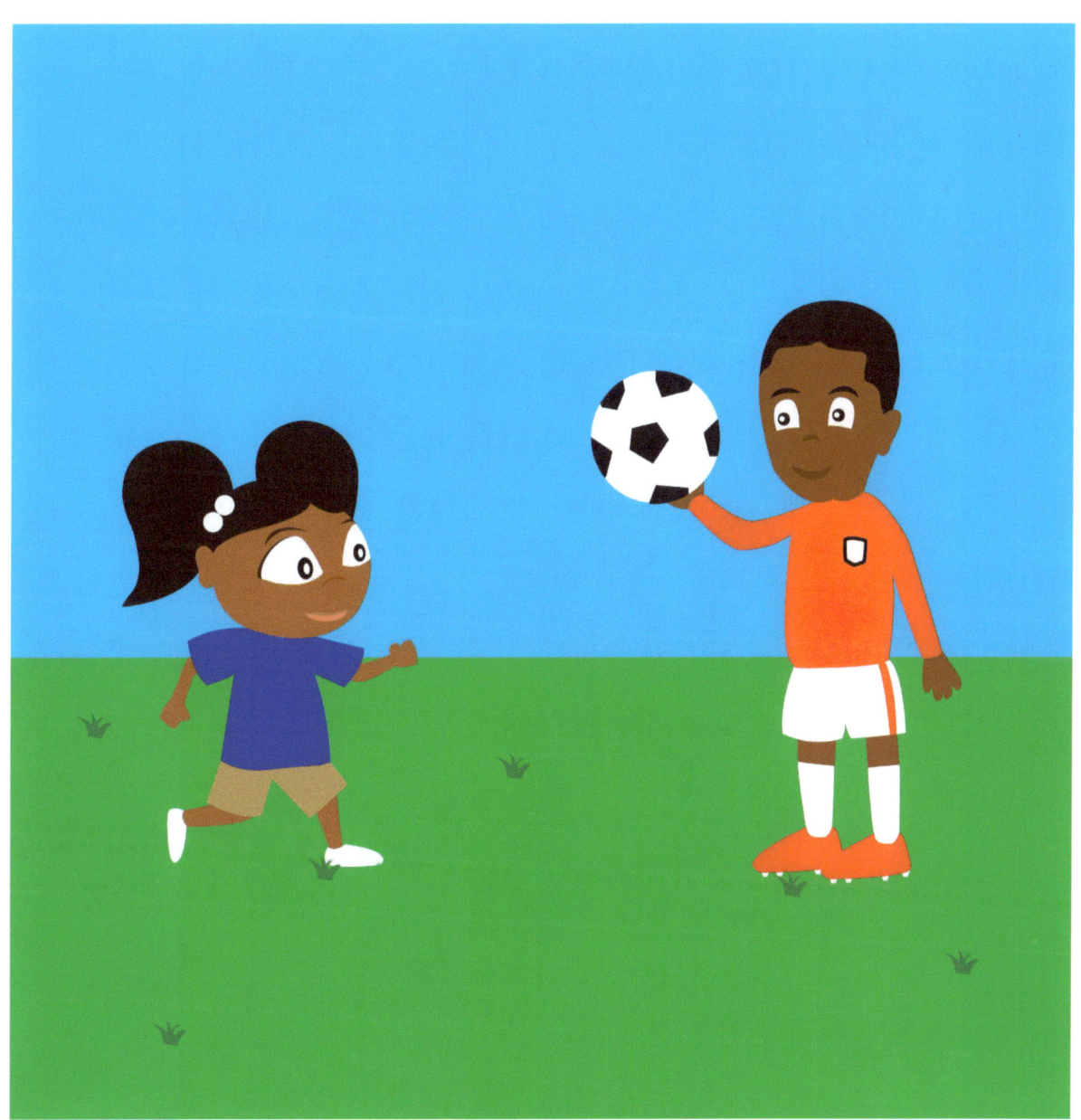

Bryce explained to Michelle, that before every game he takes his pump, which helps open his lungs. When he's resting he drinks some water and if he needs his pump he takes it again. Bryce told Michelle something that stuck with her for the rest of the day. "I don't think about my asthma during the game. It's easy, I just don't let it control me, I control it. No matter how hard it gets, I believe that this disease won't get the best of me."

For the whole week Michelle kept thinking about what her friend Bryce said. "I don't let it control me, I control it and believe in yourself while you're at it."

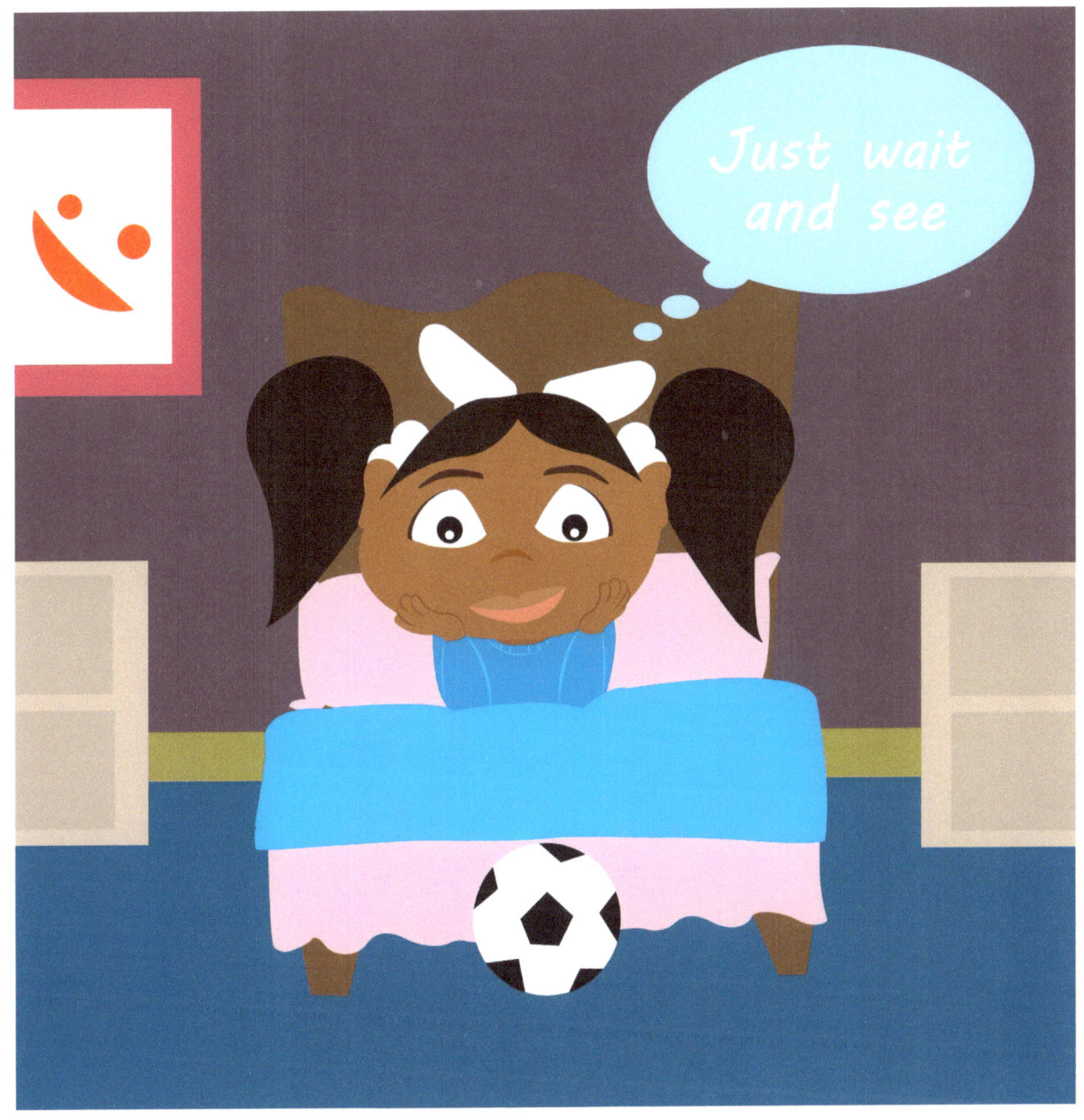

Michelle kept telling herself that whole week she was going to do this. She was going to beat this disease.

That next week at school was kickball tryouts. Michelle said to herself, this is my time, things are going to change. She picked up her inhaler, took a puff and ran to the field to show everyone what she could do.

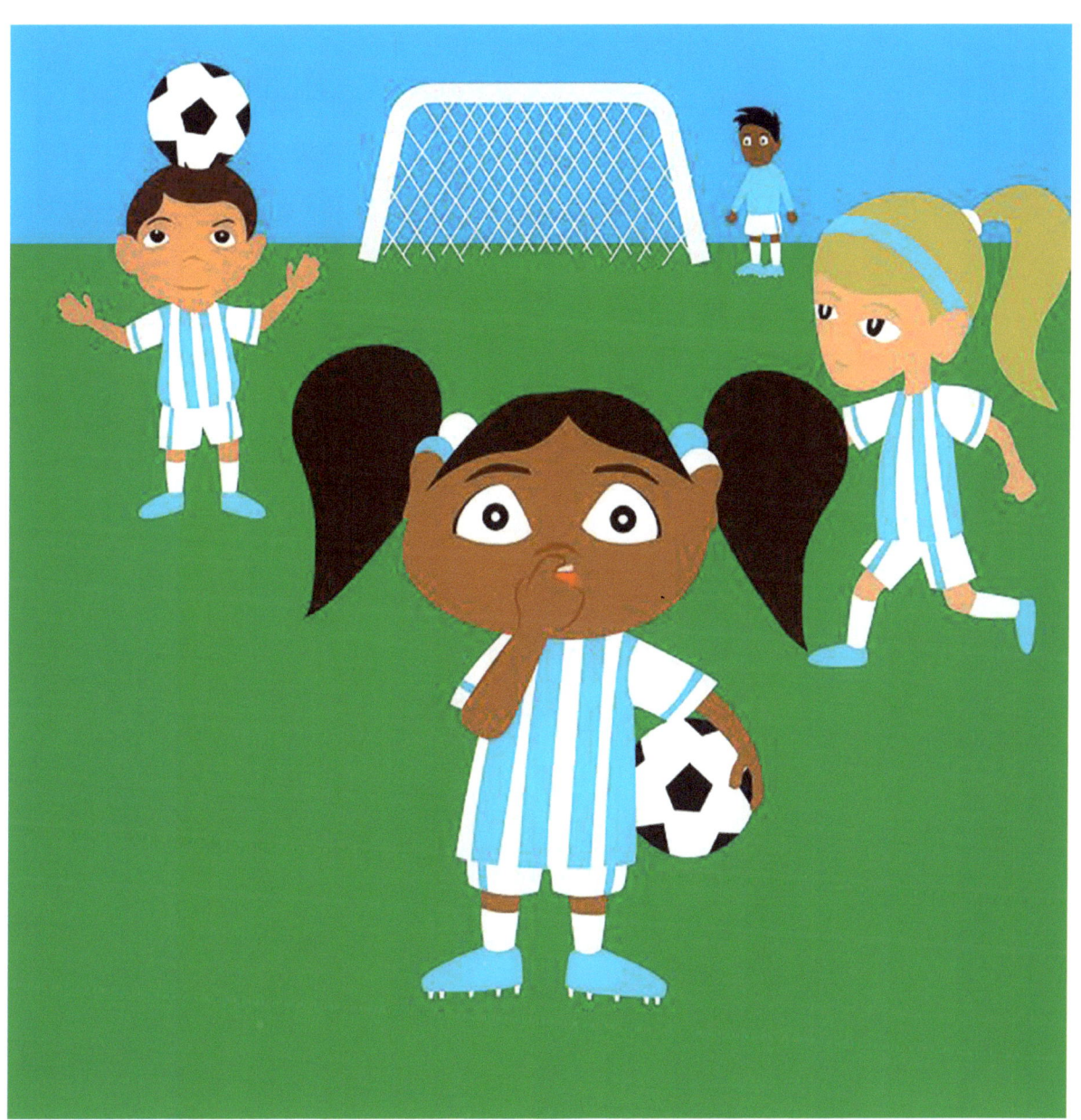

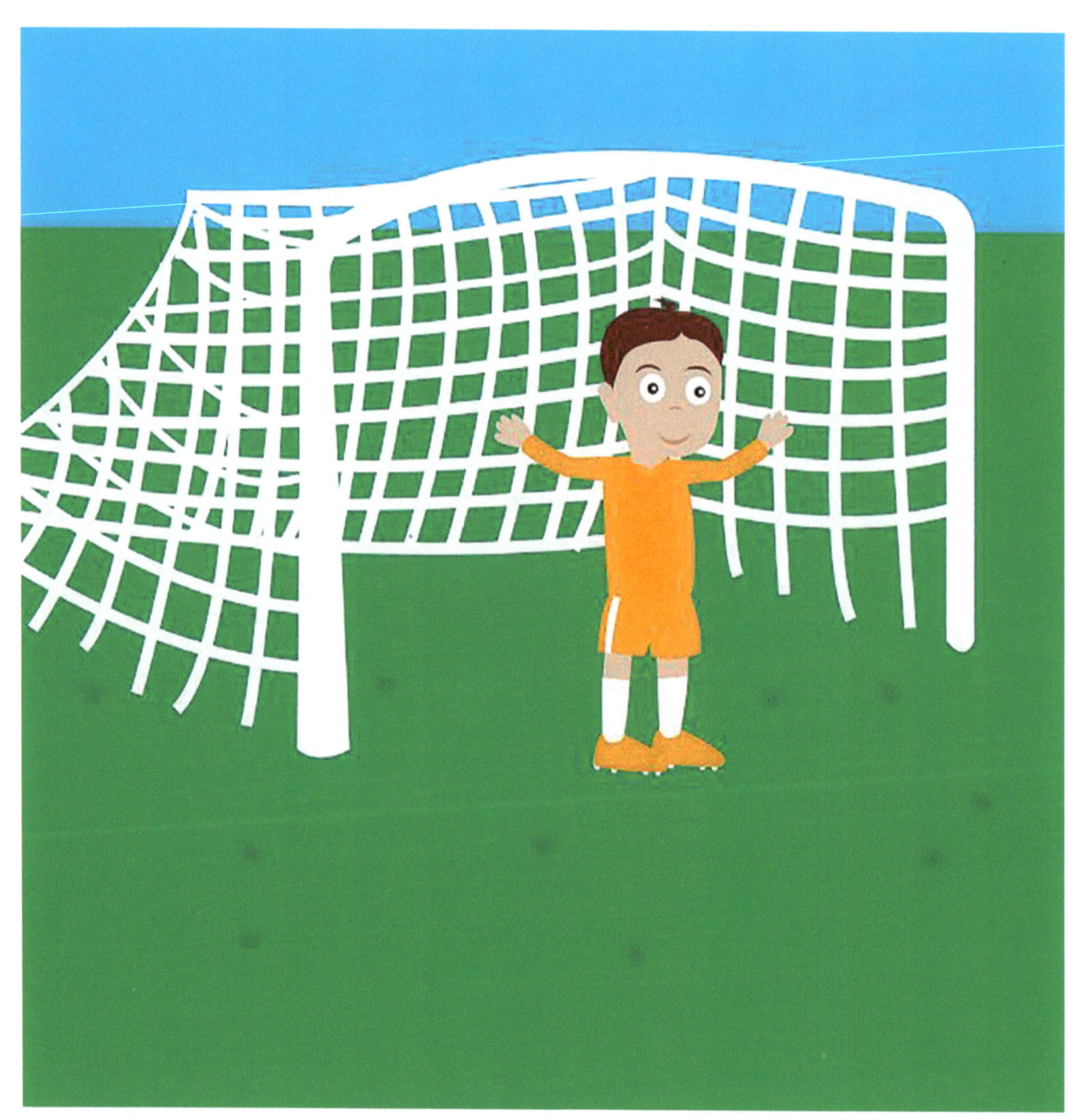

You know what happened next....

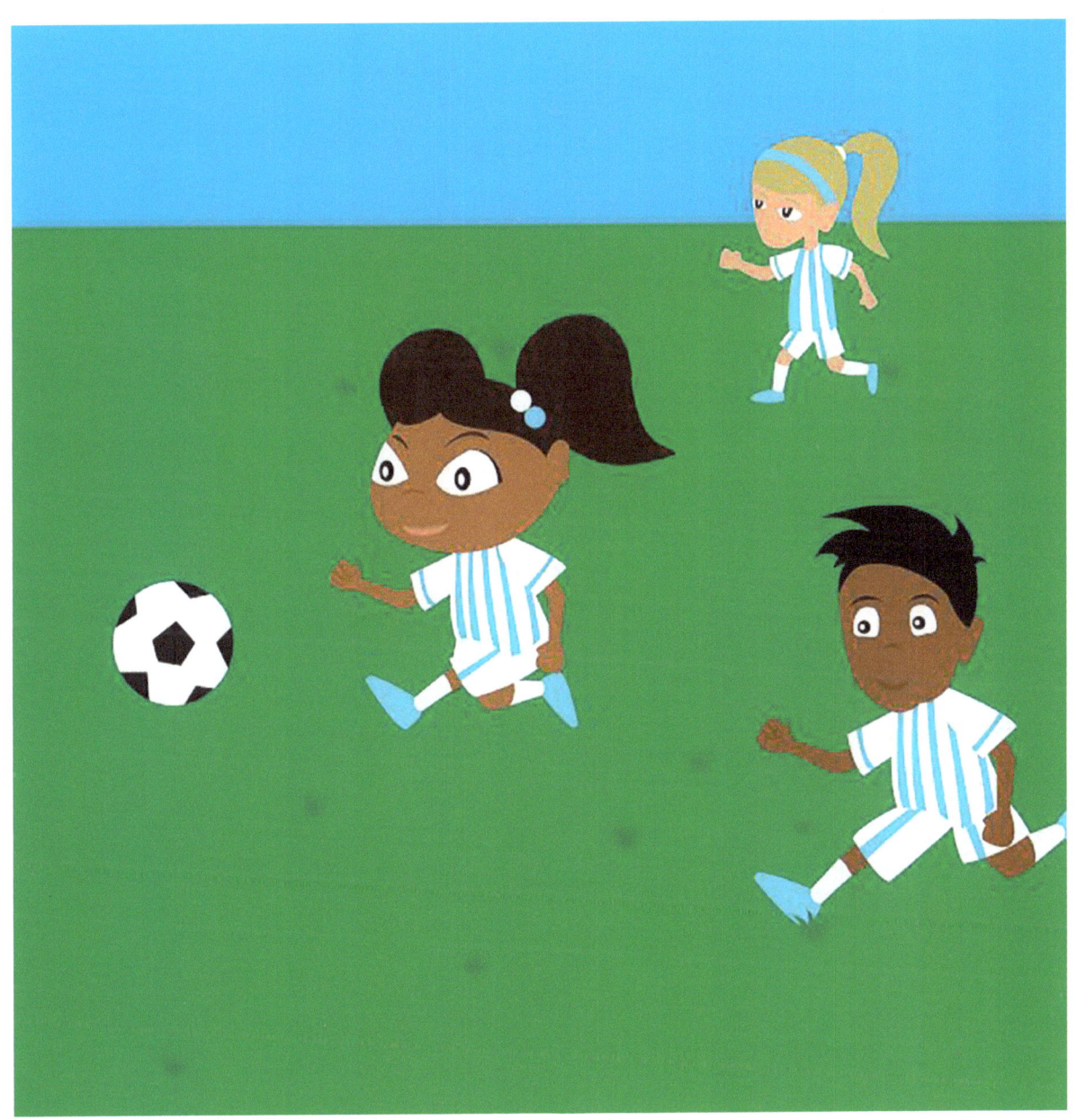

Michelle made the team. Meet the new kicker!!

Michelle finally realized that even though she has asthma, that won't stop her from enjoying her life. It may slow her down sometimes, but it won't stop her from having fun. Michelle is still the life of the party!

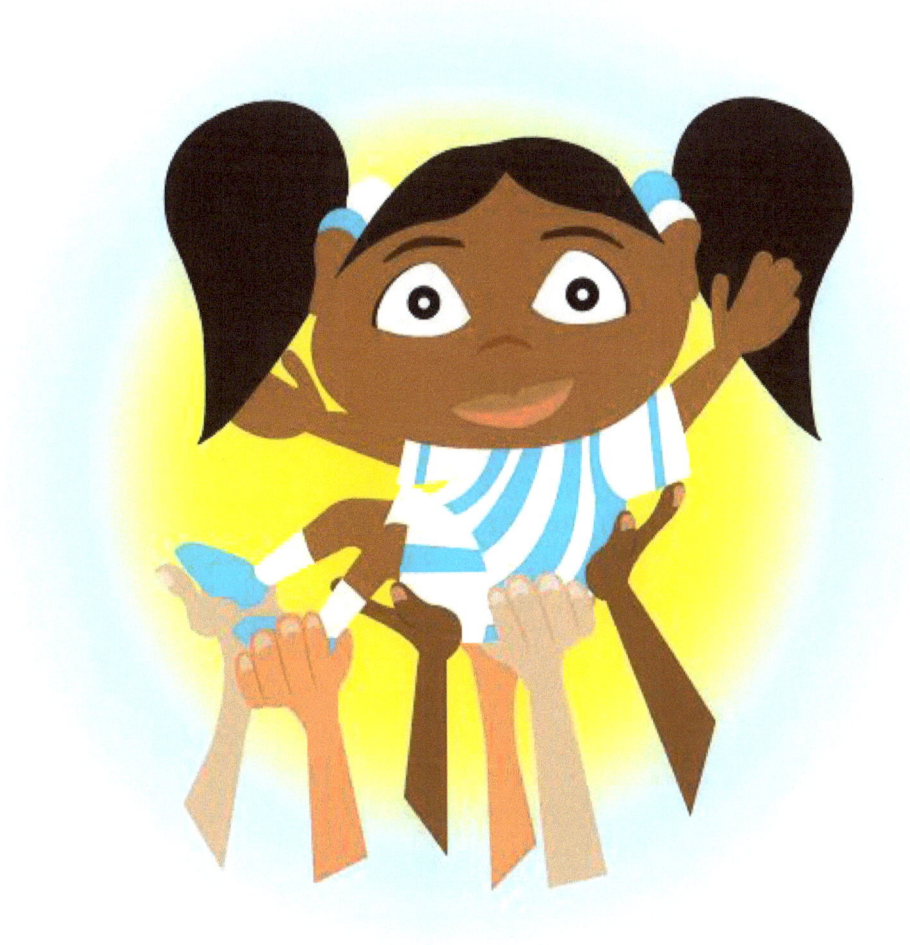

FINAL REMARKS FROM IEISHA MICHELLE

It is my greatest desire that you realize you are the expression of beautiful grace, exactly the way you are. Yet, you may have a different path to take, or face some unimaginably difficult circumstances as a child, and well on into adulthood.

I wrote this book as a voice of the young overcomer, the voiceless children who need the confidence to know that they have a purpose, and an amazing destiny to fulfill. I want kids to embrace every difference, and revel in the fact that they possess the ability, just like I found, to become the greatness they were created to be.

Please enjoy, support, and promote *The Girl with a Heart of Gold*; it just may change a child's life.

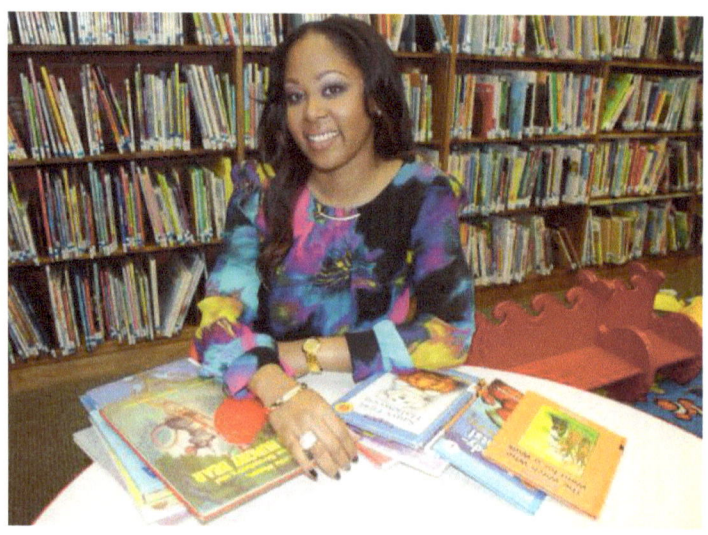

ABOUT THE AUTHOR

IEISHA MICHELLE was born in Anaheim, California on September 26, 1982. She, in her own rights, has been an inspirational and children's literature writer as long as she can remember. She would sit in her room and write, sometimes for hours, about a multitude of subjects. Writing was a way for her to express the massive amount of thoughts and creativity she sheltered in her heart. Ieisha has been a music lover, with a deep passion for the artistry of each word, as well as each note; and she credits herself as a self-proclaimed food connoisseur for the majority of her life. Looking back in Ieisha's childhood room, you will find dozens of journals where she has jotted down random thoughts, and emotions, writing whatever came to her imaginative mind. As a young adult, Ieisha Michelle pursued her education, and earned her Bachelor's Degree in Communications from the California State University of Los Angeles, and continued on to complete a Master's Degree in Entertainment Business from Full Sail University. Having a successful education, career, loving family, and an ocean of friends, she felt that there was something yet to be accomplished, and Ieisha stepped out on faith to author her first of many books, based on her own life experiences of growing up and dealing with the challenges faced by an asthmatic child.

Get In Touch

I always love to hear from my readers and supporters. Please don't hesitate to contact me at info@thegirlwithaheartofgold.com.

Connect With Us...

Please make sure to follow *The Girl with a Heart of Gold* on Facebook, Instagram and Twitter to get the latest updates and announcements.

www.ingramcontent.com/pod-product-compliance
Lightning Source LLC
Chambersburg PA
CBHW042144290426
44110CB00002B/113